MEDICINES AND DOSAGES TO CURE CORONAVIRUS

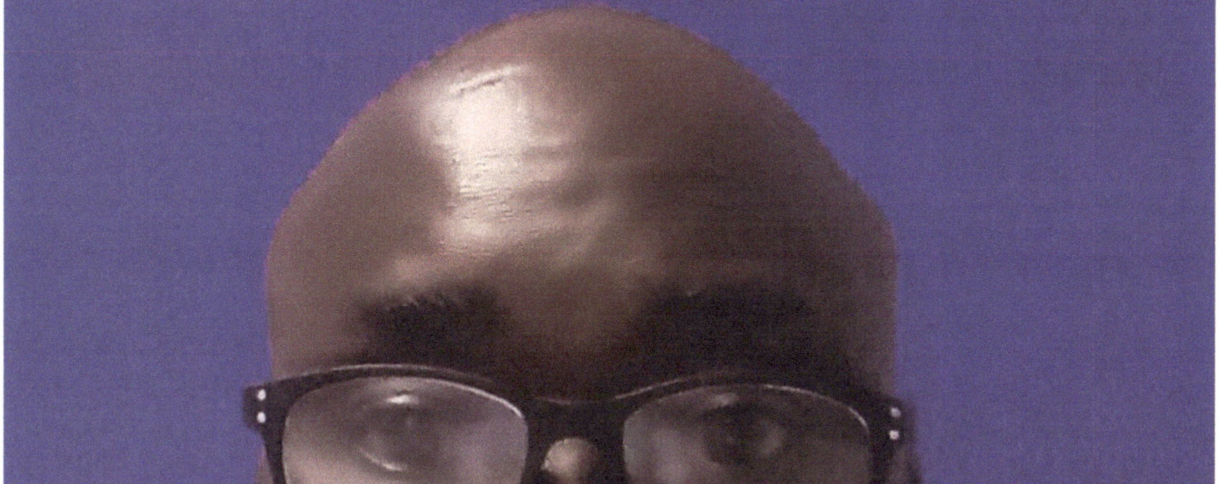

PIERRE JOUISSANCE 2020

All rights reserved. No part of this publication may be reproduced, distributed, or transmitted in any form or by any means, including photocopying, recording or other electronic or mechanical methods, without the prior written permission of the author.

US *Copyright* 2020

Second Edition

Table of Contents

1- Introduction

2- The patient's environment and medications that will be needed.

2-1 Environment

2-2 Medication

3- Preparation of bitter leaves for the patient to drink whenever thirsty.

3-1- What are the benefits of bitter leaves to make a tisane for the patient to drink whenever thirsty?

3-2- Which bitter leaf is recommended for making the tisane?

4- Tetracycline: is an antibiotic according to my experience that can treat the coronavirus. Let us say a few words about tetracycline.

4-1- How many tetracycline pills should the patient take each day? And what time of day?

5- Ampicillin: What are the symptoms for a patient to develop before giving a small ampicillin?

6- Preparation of the syrup bottle: the amount of syrup to prepare for the patient

6-1 What quantity of syrup should the patient take each day? What time of day?

6-2 List of ingredients and dosages you will need to prepare the syrup bottle

7- What foods should patients eat every day? Should the patient drink juice?

8- Castor oil: the role of castor oil. Which side of the patient's body should you pass it to?

9- Vicks: the role of Vicks. Which side should you pass it to?

10- Conclusions and recommendations

1-   Introduction

My name is Pierre R Jouissance, I live in New Jersey (USA). First, I want to apologize to the readers because I am not a perfect writer, but I write this book in order to share an important message.

The purpose of this publication is to share the good news to the world, especially to the United States. What good news is this? From today onward, people will no longer die of coronavirus, because a sick person can treat himself if he properly applies all the tips in this book. Someone can get coronavirus, but he can be treated in 3 days.

I am announcing in the name of Jesus since the publication of this document, there must be no more restrictions. Life must resume as it was before, which means it is no longer an obligation to be required to wear a mask or observe social distance. All schools, all universities must reopen without restriction. All clubs, all restaurants, all churches must resume their activities. If you get the coronavirus, you can be healed in 3 days. Jesus' people must live comfortably, and they cannot tie their faces all day long.

Everyone is asking who gives me the authority to speak like that. I will explain to you where I find authority to speak like that. The first thing I have spoken to Jesus. I told Jesus I am tired of putting a piece of cloth on my face and everything being closed. Everyone has a way Jesus answer them. The way Jesus answered me, He wrote the answers in my mind. He said to me, the fever that is hitting the world is not new, that fever has already happened in Haiti and your parents made medicine for you and God remembered all the medicine my mother called sidelia Rocher and my father called natal jouissance made for me. They gave birth to nine children and came to save all with wild leaves thanks to Jesus.

I write the list, I go to the supermarket, I buy, and I make the remedy. Now I'm not afraid of coronavirus not because I know I won't catch it. No, I can catch it, but I know how to heal right away. And that is why I want to share with the world suffering from the disease. To me, coronavirus is a simple fever, we have no reason to keep restricting.

2- The patient's environment and medications that will be needed

If you have to supervise a patient, the first thing to look for is the patient's environment, and secondly, to see if all the medications on the patient's table are in accordance with the recommendations in this document.

2-1 Environment

The patient's place should be clean. Get rid of the sick room all things that prevent him to breathe. The room should not be too cold. The patient's room temperature should be between 23 degrees Celsius to 30 degrees Celsius or 72 degrees Fahrenheit to 85 degrees Fahrenheit. If the outside temperature is not lower than 23 degrees Celsius you can open windows for patients to breathe natural air. Artificial Ventilation, fan and air conditioning are not recommended and might kill the patient. Always check the room temperature to see if it is not too cold. If the patient says he is hot and if there is no window to give the patient a little natural air : turn on the fan but make the wind hit the wall it means do not turn on the fan directly on the patient. When the patient says he is not hot, turn it off again. Whatever the reason, never turn on the air conditioning in the patient's room. I say that the corona can kill the patient if you do not follow all the contents of the book.

2-2 Medication

After you put the patient in a proper environment, this medication should be done for the patient to heal immediately.

a) Boil bitter leaves. After boiling, mix it with cool water and place it on the table. when the mixed bitter water is cool, this is the water that the patient must drink whenever he is thirsty. Please, do not give the patient cold water. Later I tell you which bitter leaves you have to to boil and how much bitter and cold water we should mix for the tisane.

b) tetracyclines 250 mg I will tell you how many pills you should give the patient per day.

c) A small ampicillin 500 mg If we see the patient coughing much later, I will tell you how many pills to give him.

d)   One bottle of syrup 750 ml Later I will tell you all ingredients needed to make the syrup.

e)   A little castor oil Later I will tell you where on the sick body to pass the oil.

f)   A little Vicks I will tell you where to put the ointment.

3-   Preparation of tisane with bitter leaves for the patient to drink whenever thirsty

To prepare the bitter tisane for the patient you will put in a pot ¼ lb of cerasee or neem and put 1 gallon of water + 2 cups of water so that when it boils to come up to a gallon.

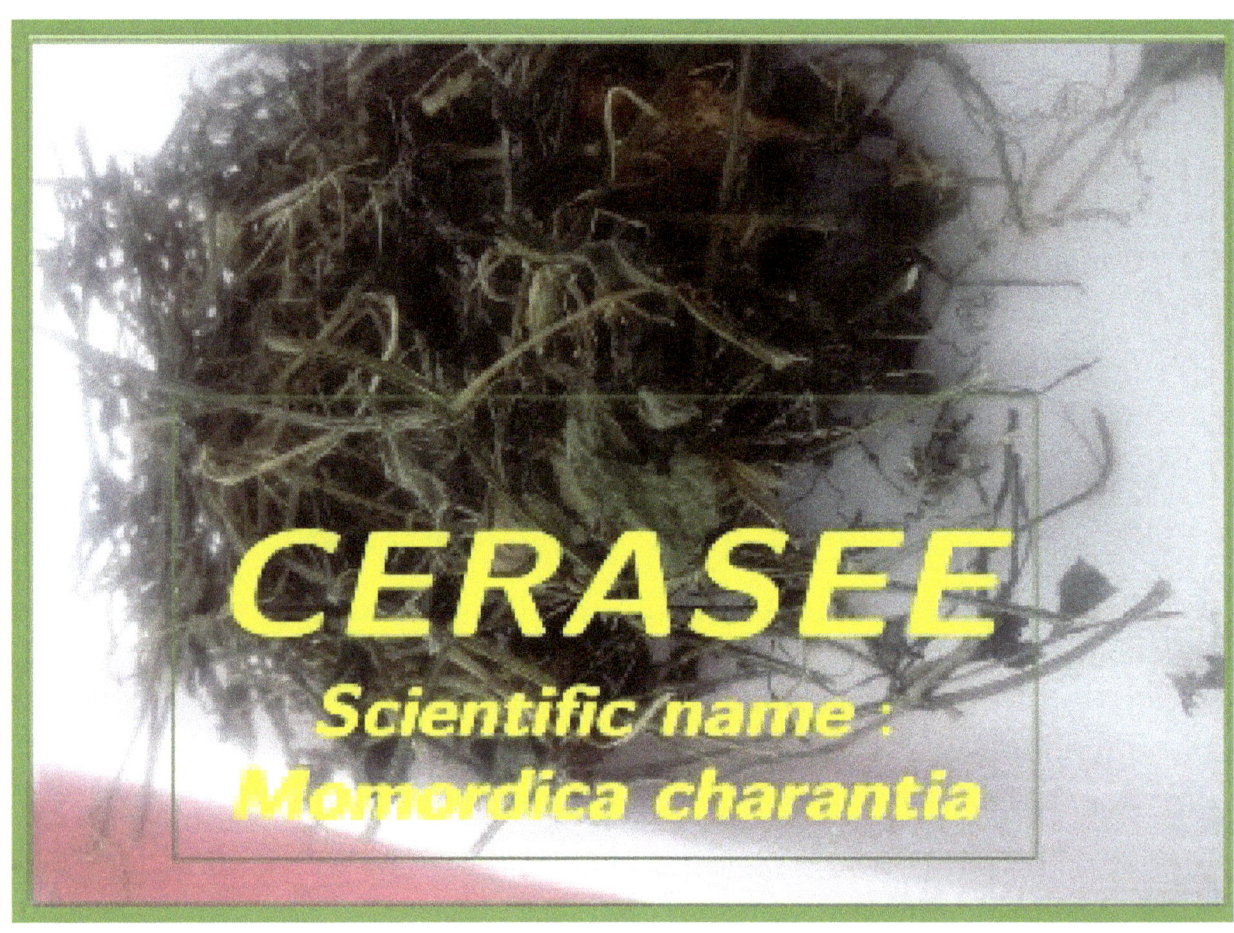

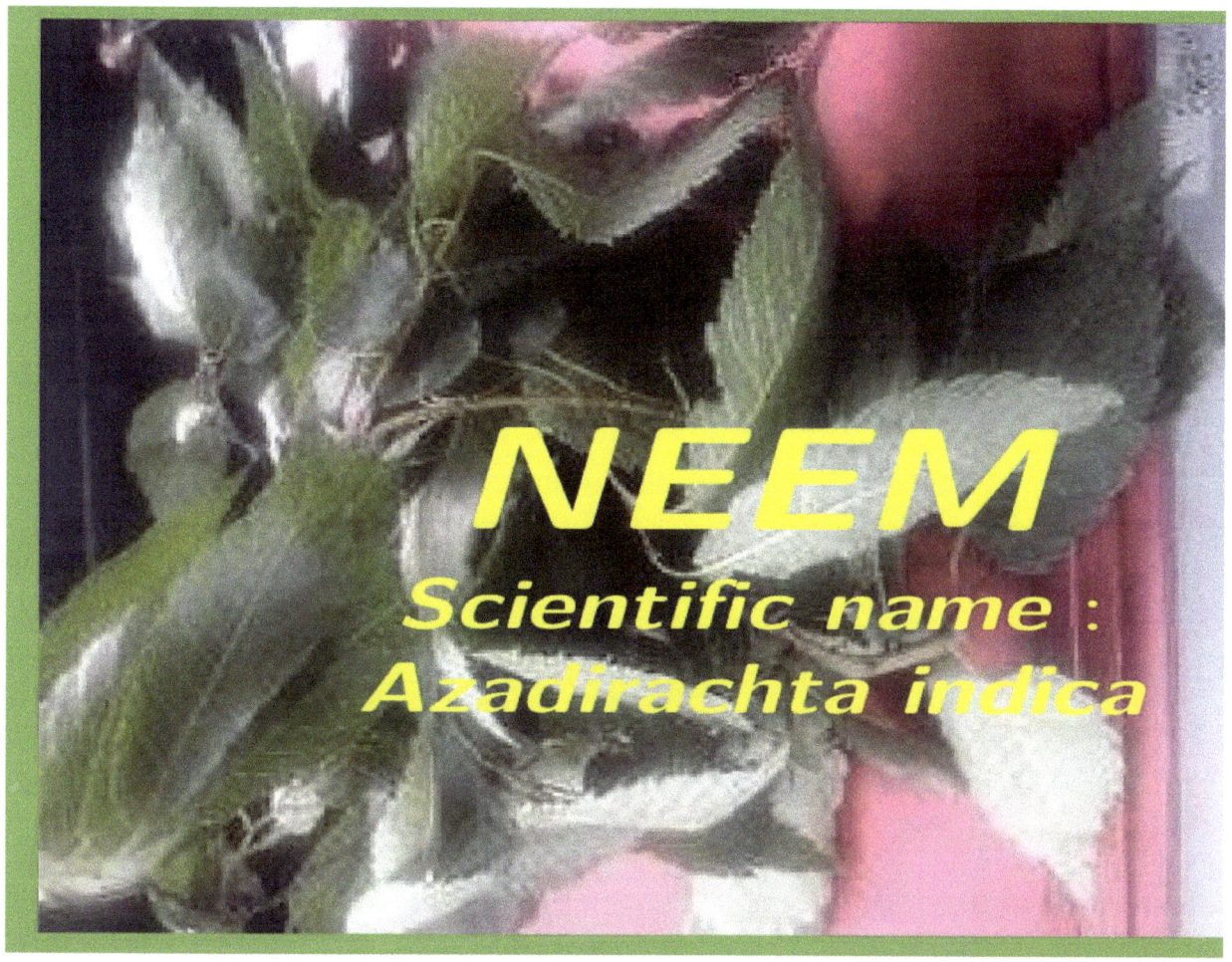

After it boils, after 4 minutes you turn the oven off and leave it to cool and then drain it with a sieve. Bitter water is called bitter concentrated water. You cannot give the patient concentrated water because it is too strong. The patient has to drink bitter water with 50% concentrated mixed with 50% ordinary water. I call ordinary water the water you use to drink when you are not sick. This means, to give the patient bitter water when he is thirsty, you will mix one gallon of ordinary water with one gallon of concentrated water and this will give you 2 gallons. We call this new product (2 gallons): mixed bitter water. This is the water that the patient drinks when he is thirsty. This water must be cool and not frozen, the temperature of the water for the patient to drink can be between 19 degrees Celsius to 21 degrees Celsius or between 65 degrees Fahrenheit to 75 degrees Fahrenheit. Anyway, you got some experience in tropical countries when you open your pipe, the water has a temperature, the mixed bitter water you give the patient must have the same temperature. That means the bitter mixed water must be cool but not frozen. The patient should eat sometimes salted foods to be thirsty. The rest of the mixed bitter water can be stored for tomorrow because it can be kept for 48 hours. After 48 hours you must boil another tisane. However, if you have a refrigerator it can take more days but be sure to remove it from the refrigerator early to defrost it because you should not give the patient iced water. When a person is sick, he would like the concentrated bitter water and the mixed bitter water to be available.

We would like some big companies to launch in the production of these bitter waters on the market. They can pasteurize the bitter water so that it can be kept for several days. But caution, we do not recommend for these big companies to go into artificial products. They must be made from natural leaves and all standards must be respected to make these bitter waters.

3-1- What are the benefits of bitter leaves to make the tisane for the patient to drink whenever thirsty?

The scientific name of the bitter leaf in general is Momordica Charantia. There are many chemical constituents in bitter leaf. These constituents found inside the bitter leaf are antiparasitic and antiviral.

Don't forget that, since the coronavirus enters your bloodstream, if your immune system is not strong, it will kill you. The people you see escaping are people with a good immune system. With bitter water, even if the human system is not strong, the bitter leaf has strong soldiers to attack the coronavirus. For example, the bitter leaf contains folic acid, It contains calcium, Coronavirus will break your limbs; bitter leaves will stand strong to repair your limbs. Bitter leaves have zinc: Corona makes you unable to taste anything, coronavirus makes you smell nothing; bitter leaves say no it restores the zinc correctly. He also has many other soldiers set up to deal with corona such as potassium, cobalt, copper, iron, vitamins A, C and K.

When you have corona, you drink ordinary water. Corona is happy and it multiplies quickly but when you drink bitter water mixed every time you are thirsty; corona does not find space to reproduce. Some people with corona drink bitter tea and then drink ordinary water after drinking bitter tea. This is a big mistake. Ok it's good the person took his bitter tea, because you stop corona for a little time. The fact that he drank ordinary water behind the bitter tea is as if he had washed his hands and wiped it on the floor because since you are in ordinary water your door is open for corona to live in your cells. That is why I also propose people with corona to drink bitter water mixed as drinking water when thirsty. He must drink it permanently until he is healed, and it will take only 3 days to be healed. After healing completely, he can return to ordinary water as he wishes. I announce that a person can get corona several times, but you know what to do now to heal.

3-2 Which bitter leaf is recommended for making the tisane? 2 bitter leaves I have particularly good experience with are the cerasee and neem scientific name of cerasee is Momordica M. charantia

Scientific name of neem is azadirachta indica

These 2 leaves are everywhere and are cheap, I have already given dosage for the use of these leaves.

3-3- When during the day should the patient drink the tisane?

He doesn't have time to drink the tisane. The patient must drink the tisane when he is thirsty and if he doesn't drink it he won't be cured. He does not need to drink it if he is not thirsty, so he must eat some salted foods in order to be thirsty. In the food chapter I will give you more details.

4- Tetracycline is an antibiotic according to my experience that can treat the coronavirus. Let's say a few words about tetracycline.

According to some research on tetracycline and in my experience, tetracycline is one of the best antibiotics that can act on many types of infections. Tetracycline can do coronavirus nothing by itself but when he puts together with the 2 other medicines namely the bitter water mixed with the syrup Tetracycline shows it is highly effective in coronavirus treatment. We see this when we see the patients is cured with the treatment that I propose.

4-1- How many tetracycline pills should the patient take each day? And what time of day should he take?

The patient should take tetracycline immediately in the morning, noon, and night. Take 2 pills in the morning after eating. Take 3 medications at the same time: the syrup, Bitter mixed water and the tetracycline.

After breakfast at 6 o'clock in the morning he can take a soup with bananas and meat. After the soup give the patient some small piece of fried salted herrings with bread so that he can be thirsty. He will put 4 tablespoons of syrup in a cup and he will drink 2 pills of tetracycline. After drinking the pill with the syrup, that will excite him to drink the mixed bitter water. I am sure he will be thirsty and can drink 2 glasses of mixed bitter water, and he will lie down. If the fever is high and his nose is closed, he cannot breathe, put a little castor oil and a little viscous ointment in the middle of his head. At noon you will do the same thing after eating. You do the same at night. Never forget to give the medicine to the patient 3 times a day.

5-   Ampicillin: What are the symptoms for a patient to develop before giving a small ampicillin?

I do not anticipate ampicillin in treatment. Here are the symptoms you can observe on the patient before giving him a small amount of ampicillin: Some patients with corona have a severe cough.

Since he has a cough, before you start treatment with tetracycline, after eating you put 4 tablespoons of syrup in a cup and do not give him tetracycline. You give him 2 pills of ampicillin and the syrup at 6 o'clock in the morning. Before noon if the cough does not stop, give him 2 more ampicillin pills at noon with the syrup and the bitter water. If it does not stop at 6 o'clock in the evening you give him 2 more pills. Watch for the night to see if the cough will not stop. If the cough stops now you start treatment with tetracycline. I have already explained everything to you about the treatment with tetracycline. Once you give him the ampicillin to stop the cough, do not give him ampicillin anymore. Start treatment with the tetracycline. Only give him the ampicillin to block the cough. If you see that even though you give him 2 pills of ampicillin in the morning 2 pills of ampicillin at noon 2 pills of ampicillin in the night the cough does not stop tomorrow bring the patient see a doctor to do a tuberculosis test because this book treats coronavirus only. I do not write this document to treat other diseases.

6-   Preparation of the syrup bottle: the amount of syrup to prepare for the patient

6-1   What quantity of syrup should the patient take each day? What time of day?

The amount of syrup we plan to prepare for a patient is a 750 ml bottle containing ingredients for storage for all the days the patient will need it. You will not need to put it in the refrigerator. The syrup expires in about 4 months.

You give the patient 4 tablespoons in the morning in a cup to drink with the pill. At noon you will give it the same value and at night you will give it the same value If the patient has a sore throat more than 4 tablespoons in the morning 4 tablespoons at noon 4 tablespoons in the evening , every 1 hour give him 1 teaspoon for the sore throat.

6-2   List of ingredients and dosages you will need to prepare the syrup bottle

To prepare a 750 ml bottle of syrup you will need

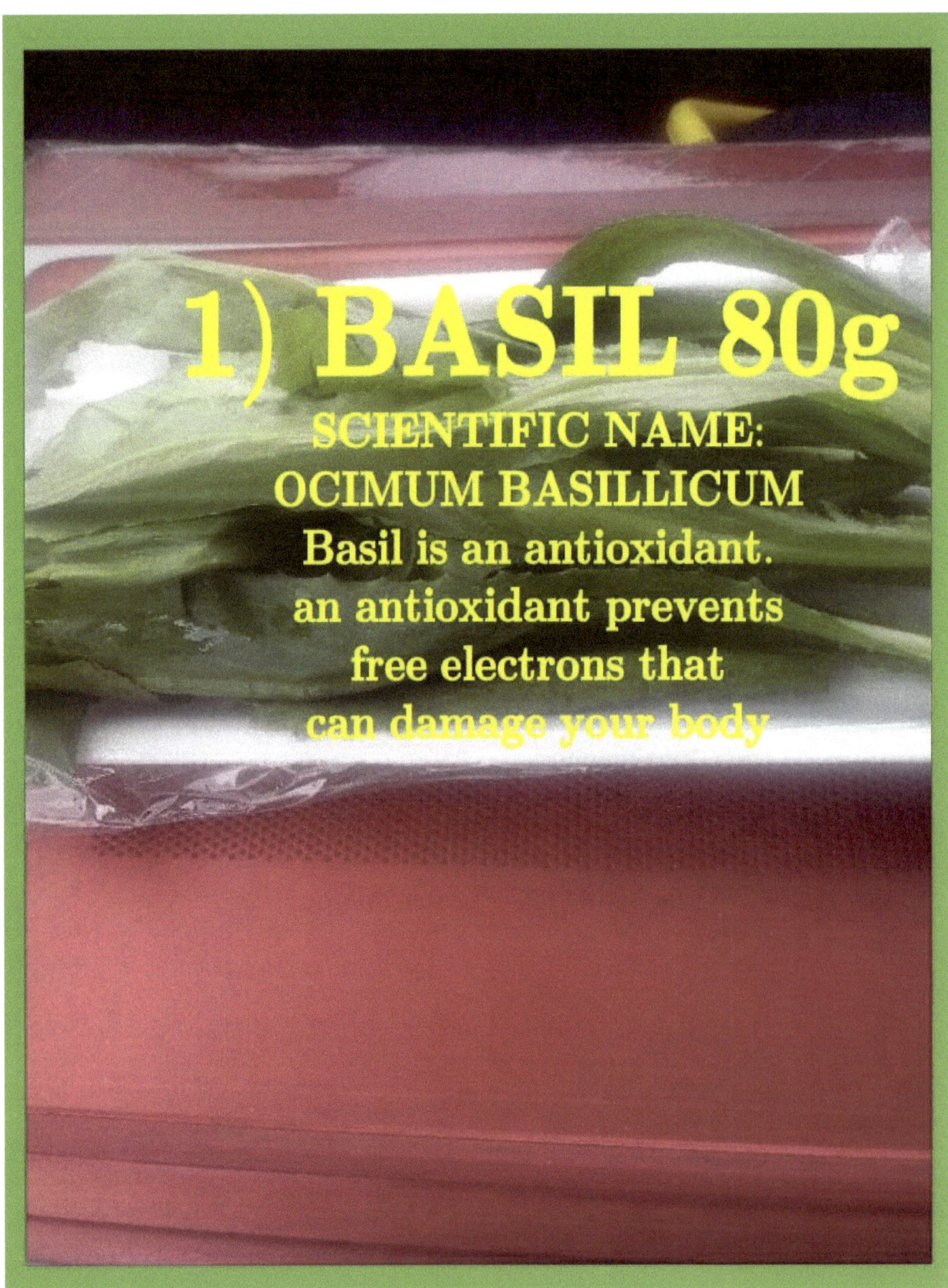

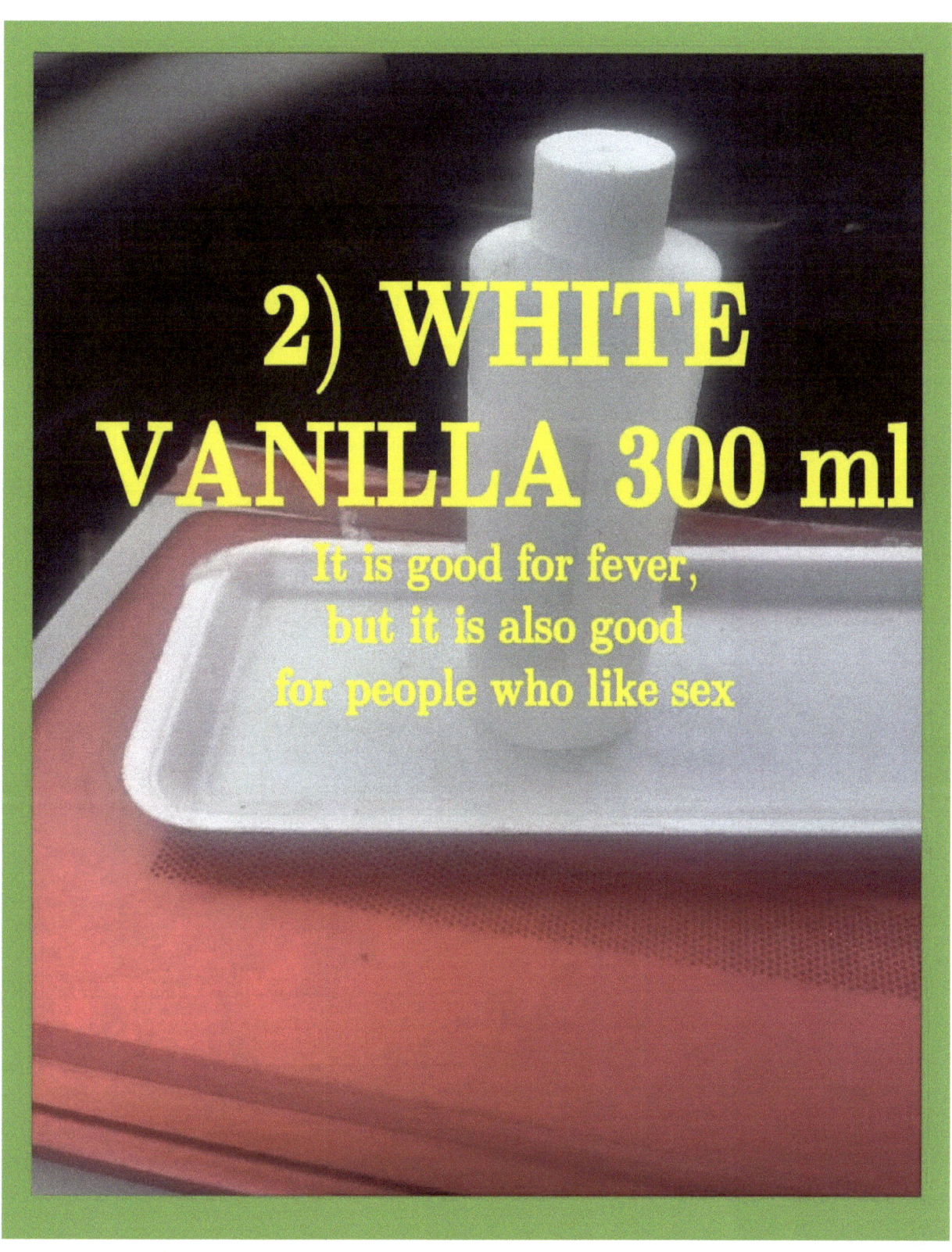

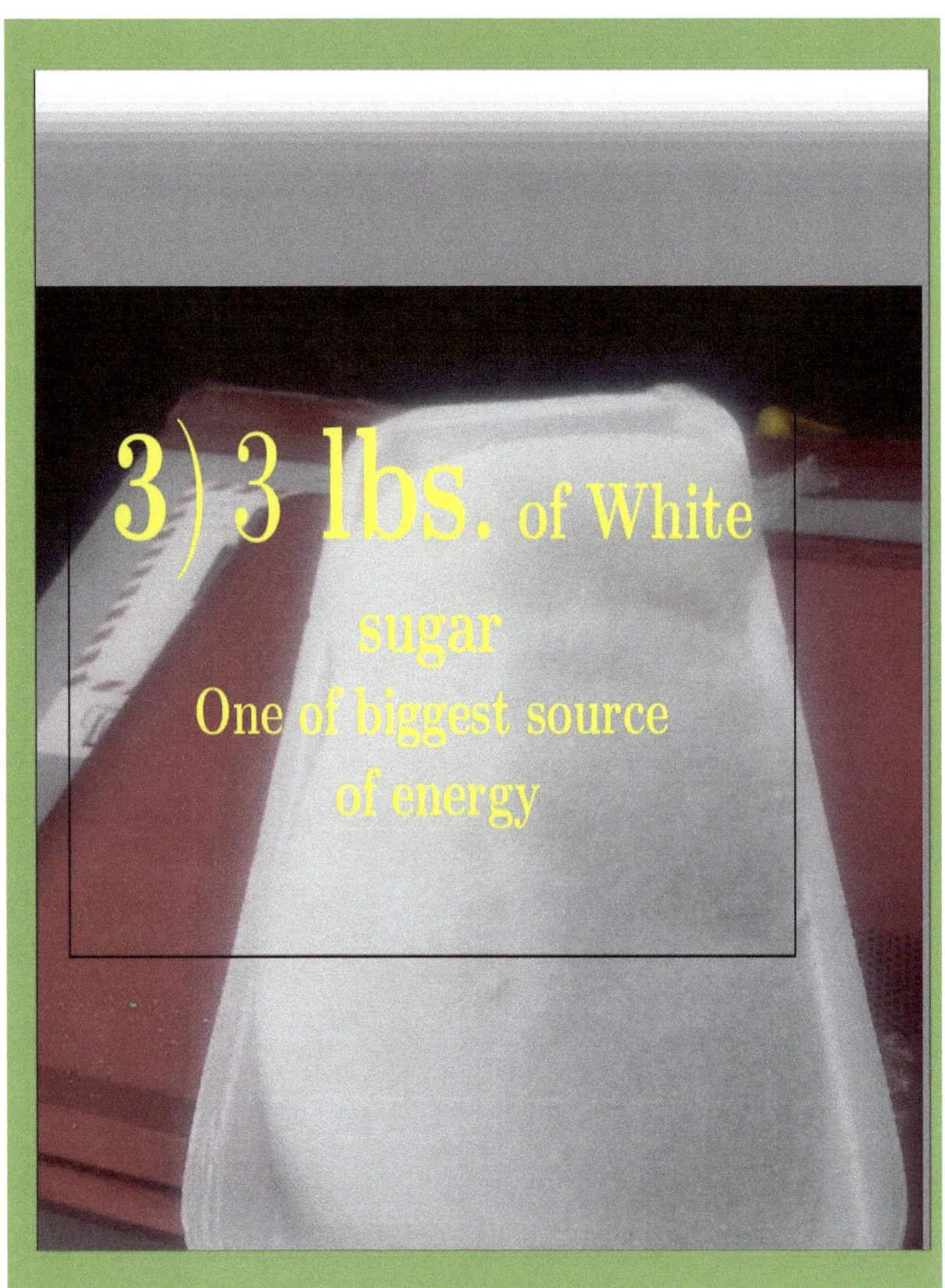

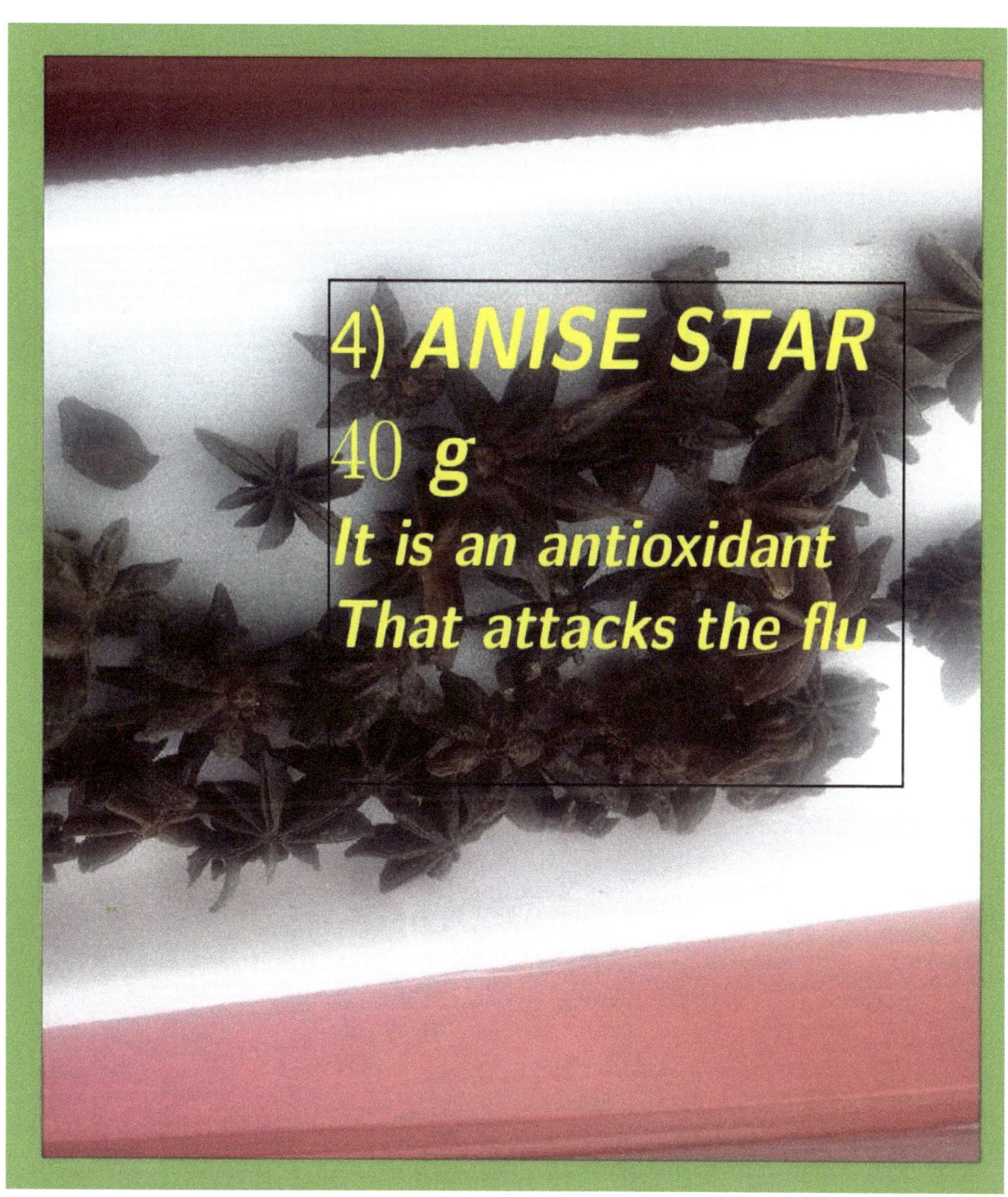

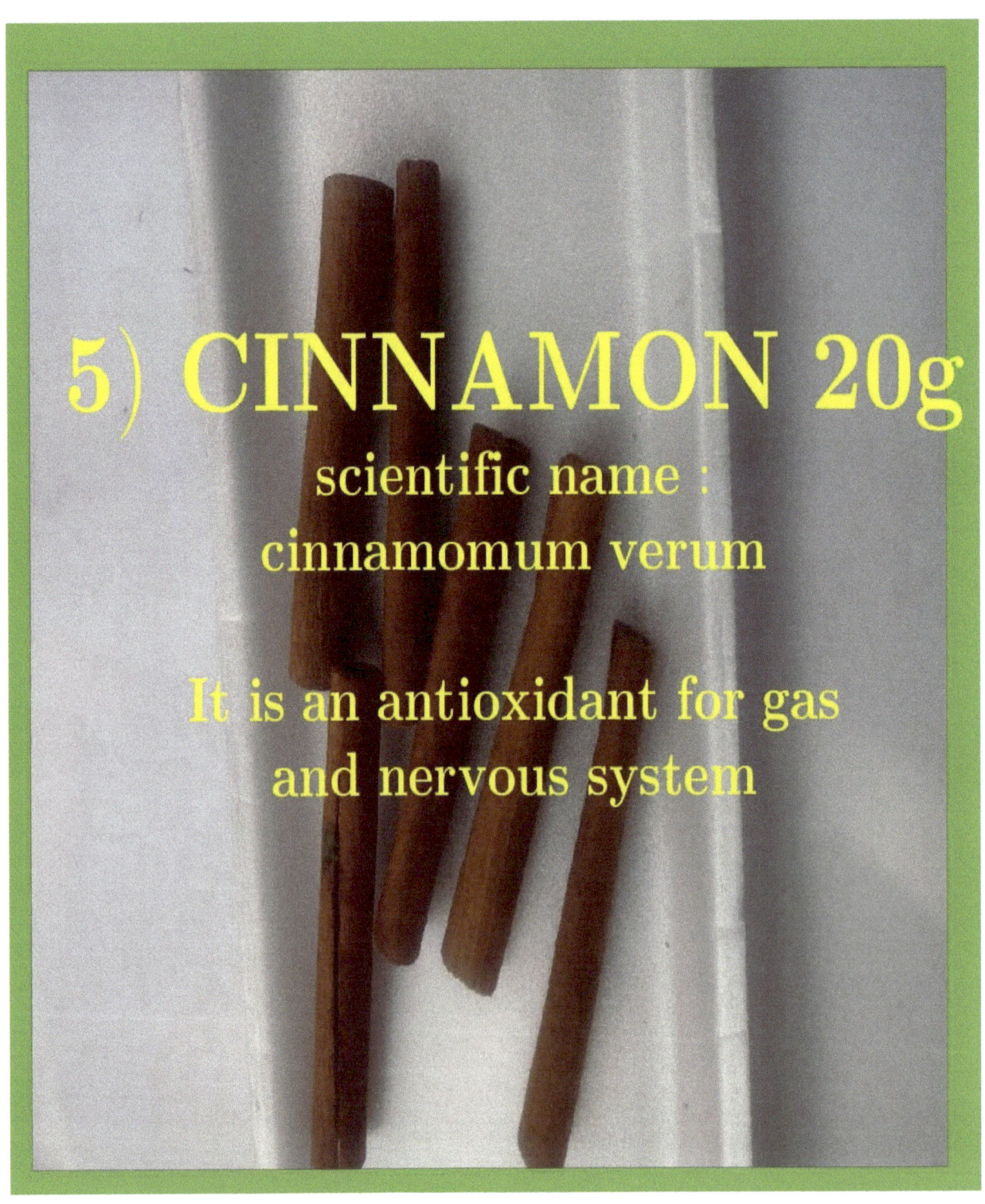

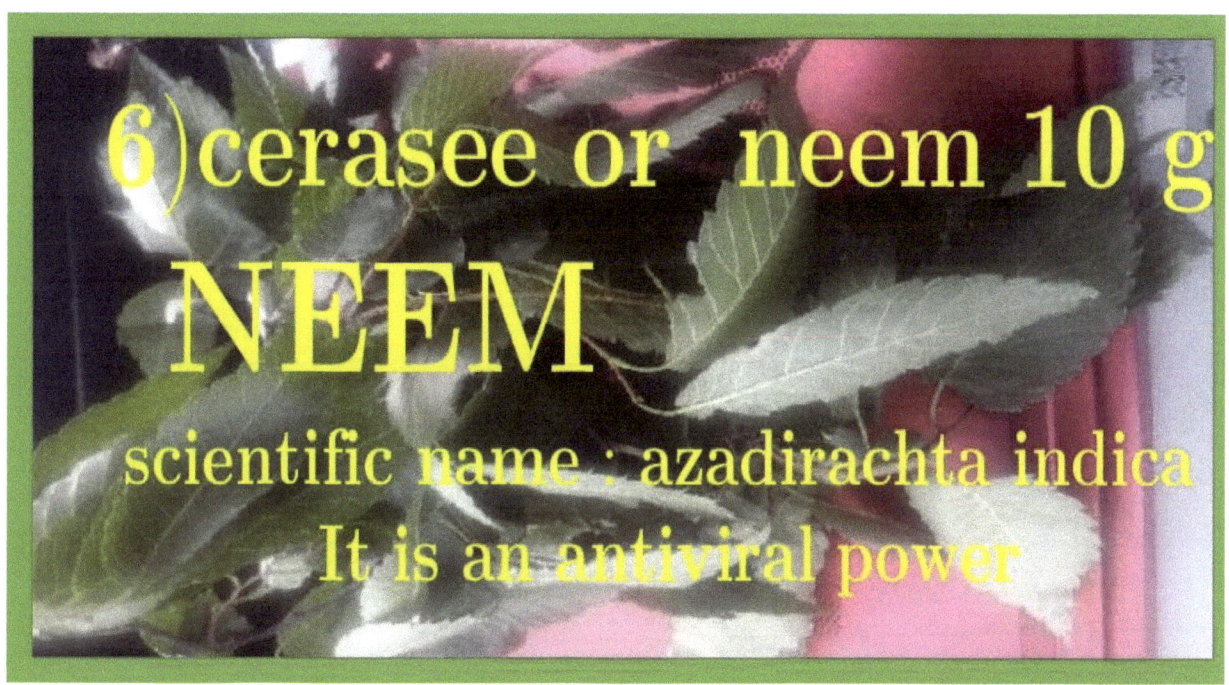

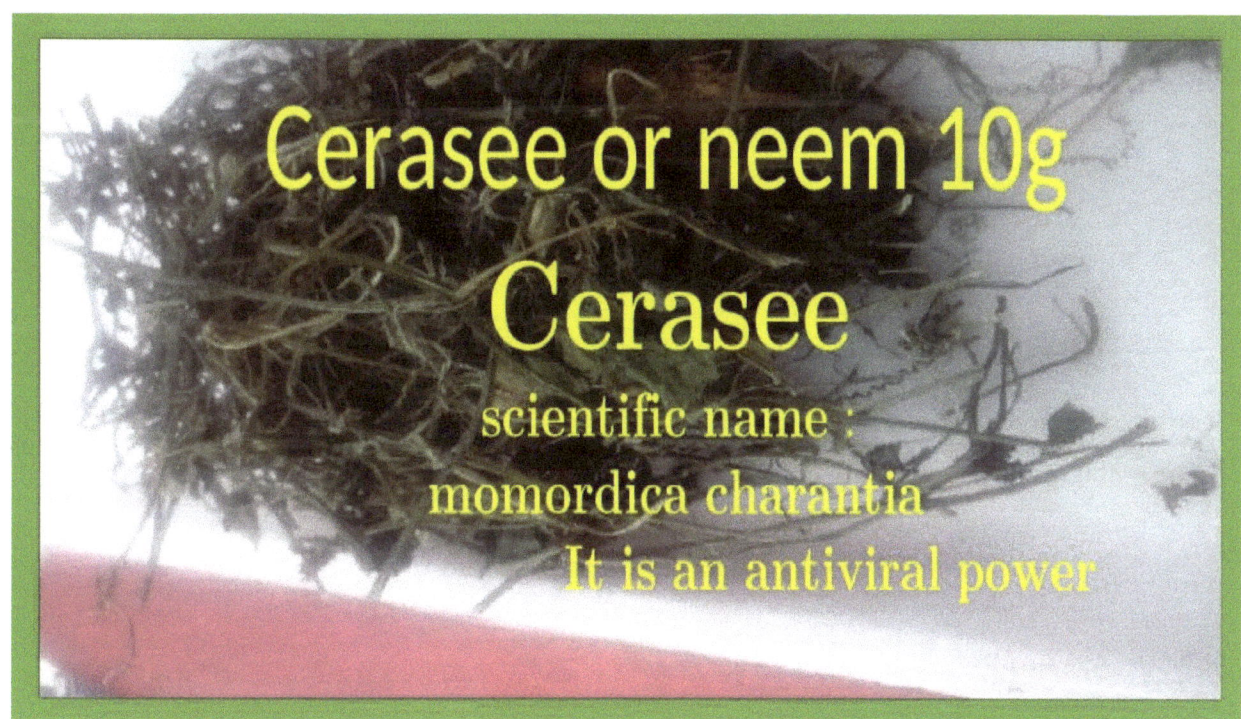

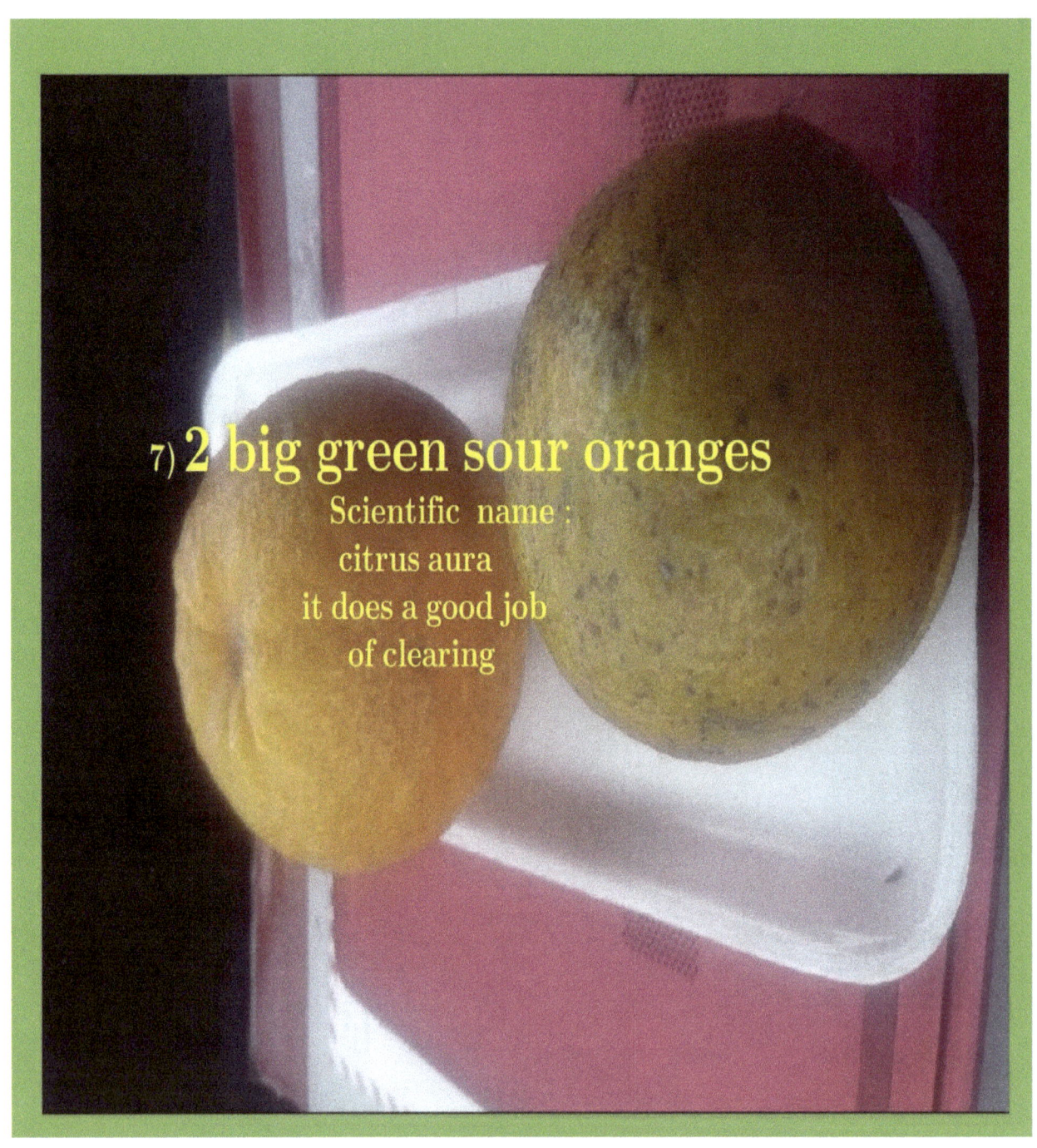

7) **2 big green sour oranges**
Scientific name :
citrus aura
it does a good job
of clearing

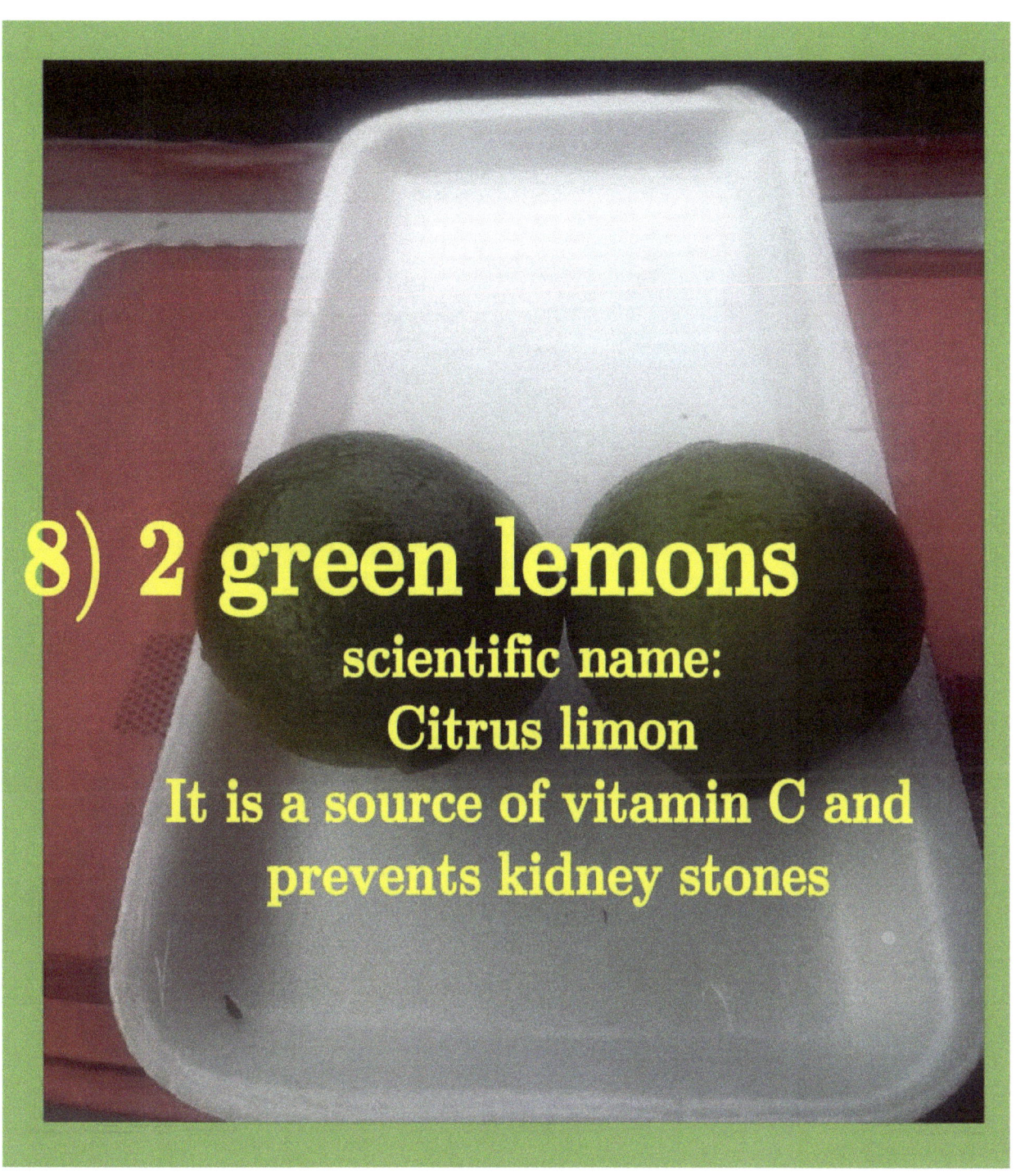

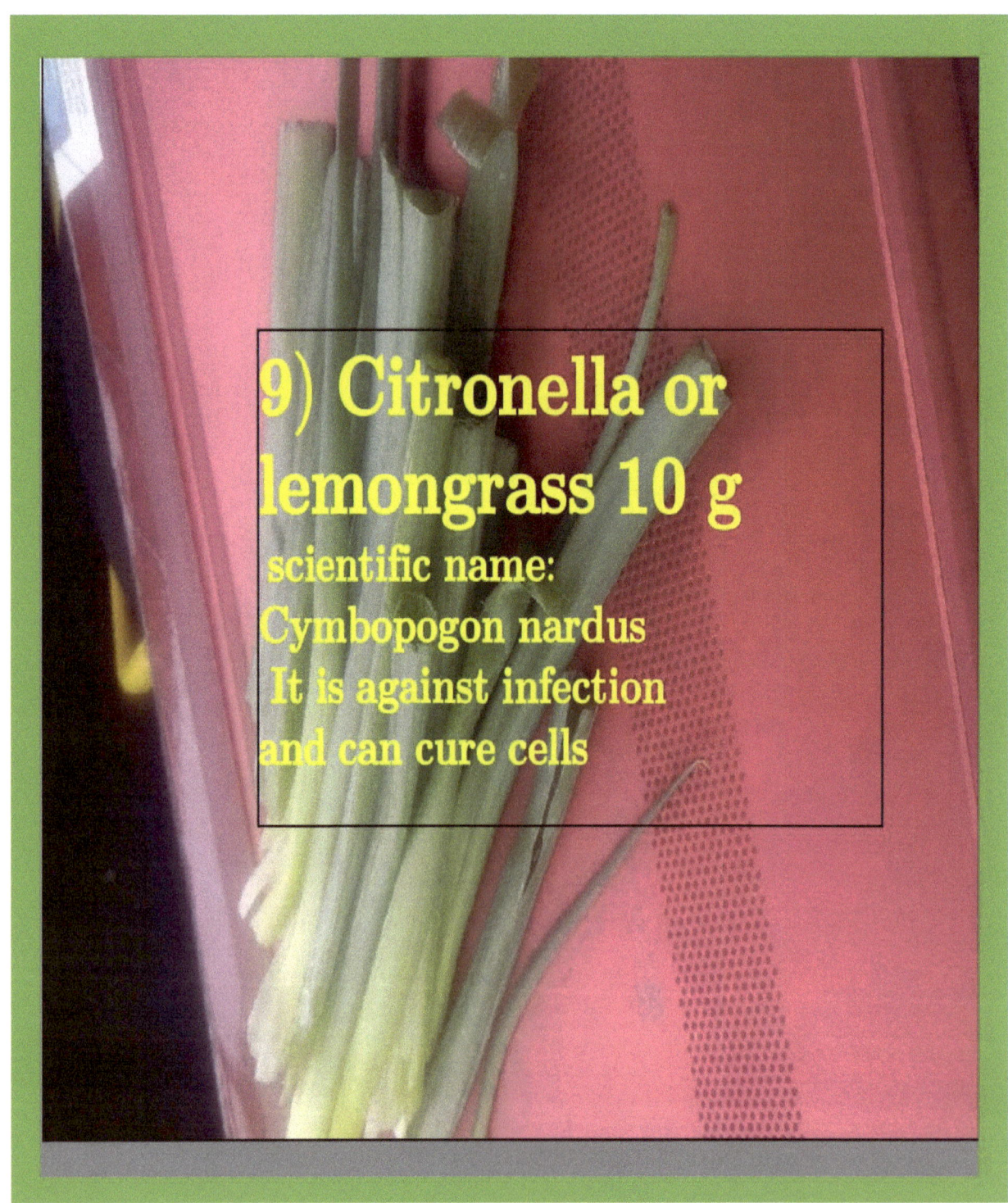

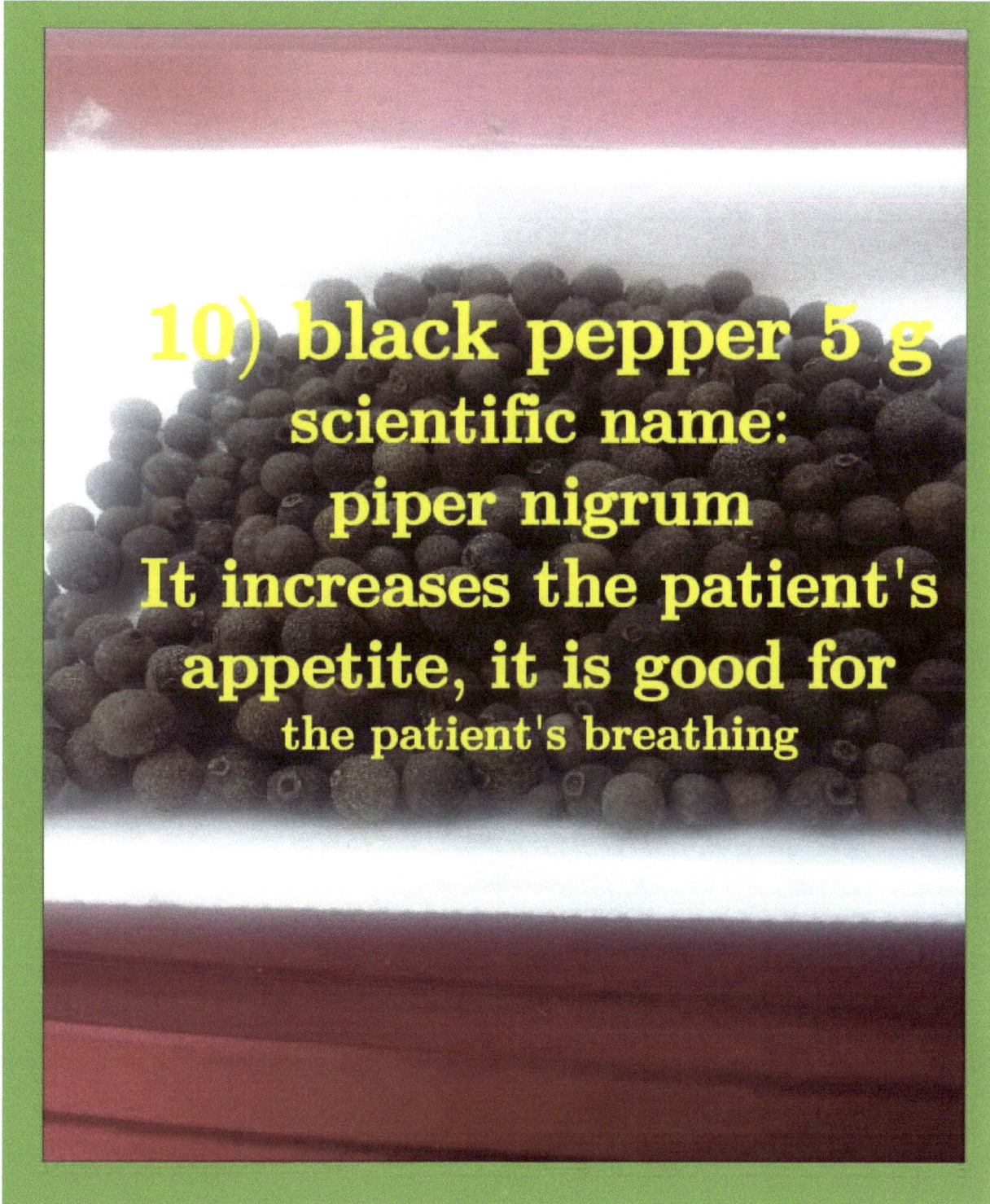

10) black pepper 5 g
scientific name: piper nigrum
It increases the patient's appetite, it is good for the patient's breathing

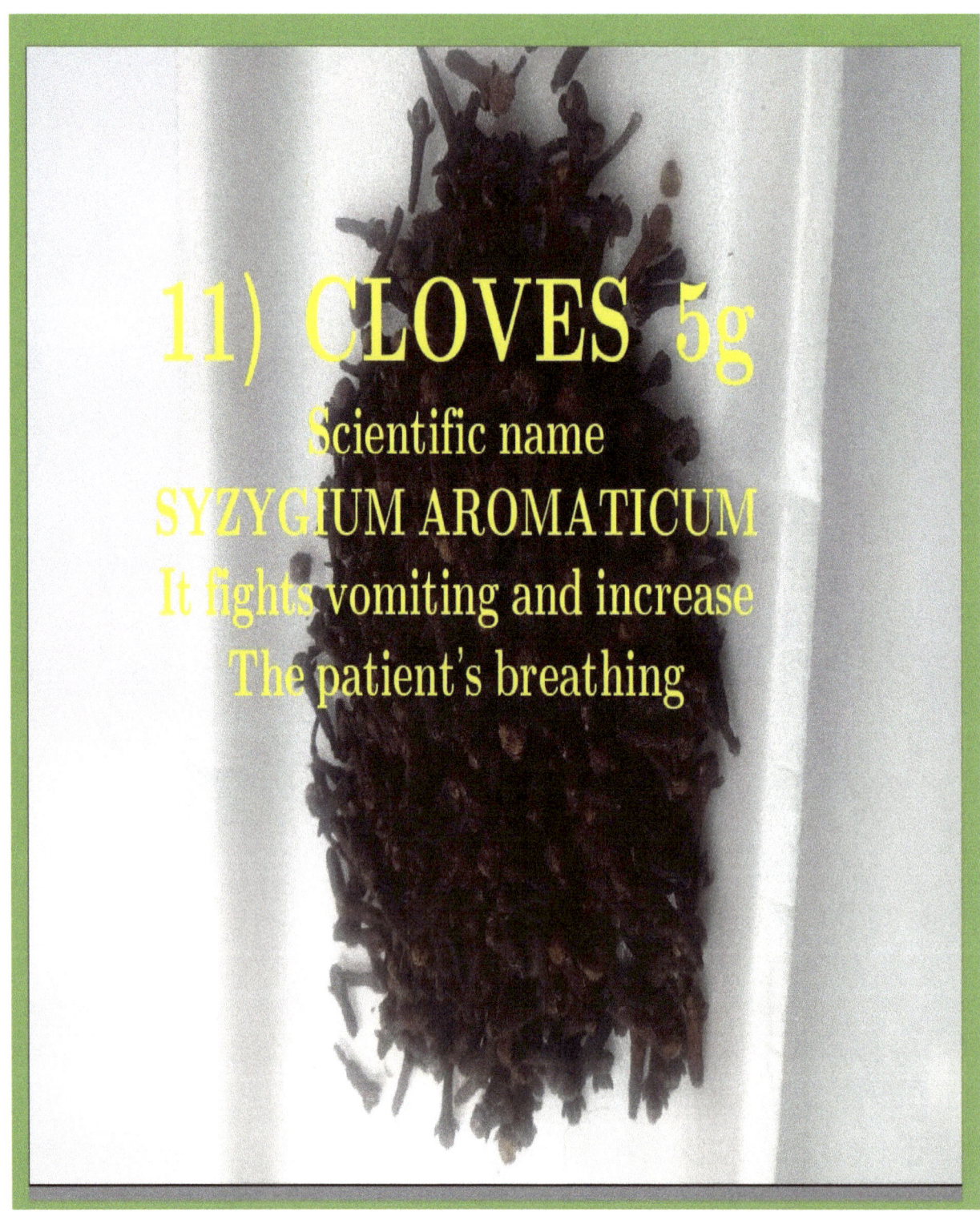

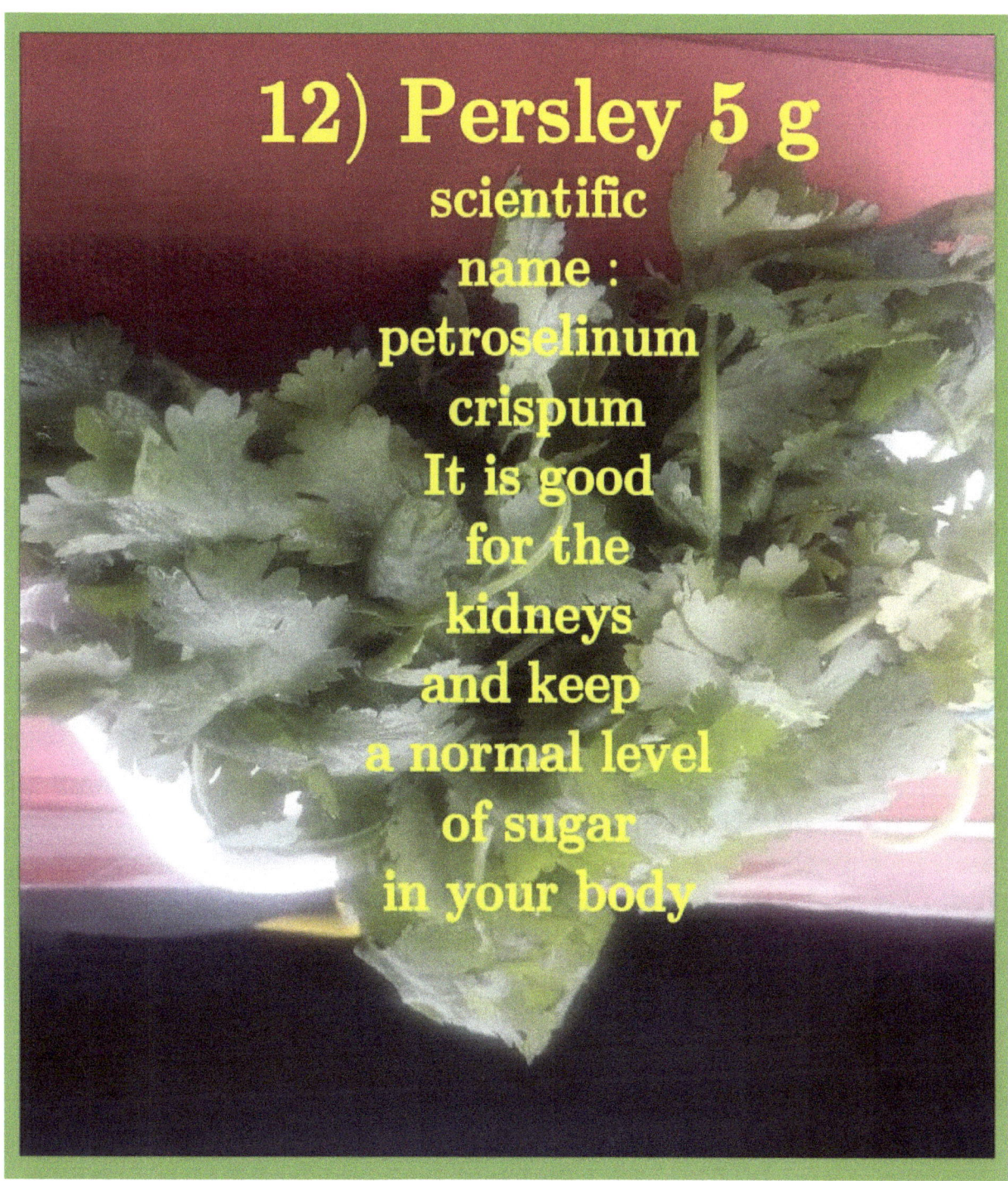

12) Persley 5 g

scientific name : petroselinum crispum
It is good for the kidneys and keep a normal level of sugar in your body

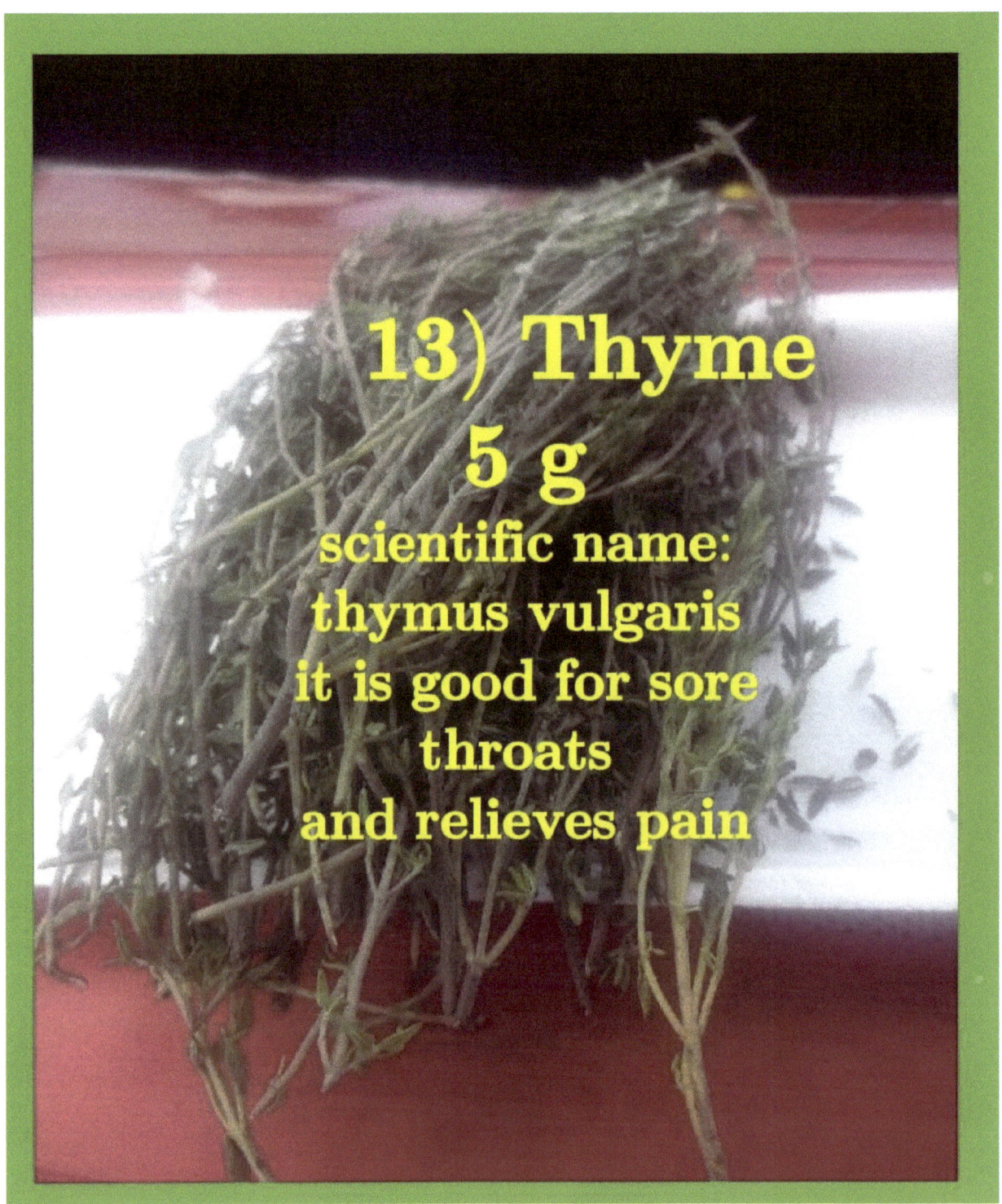

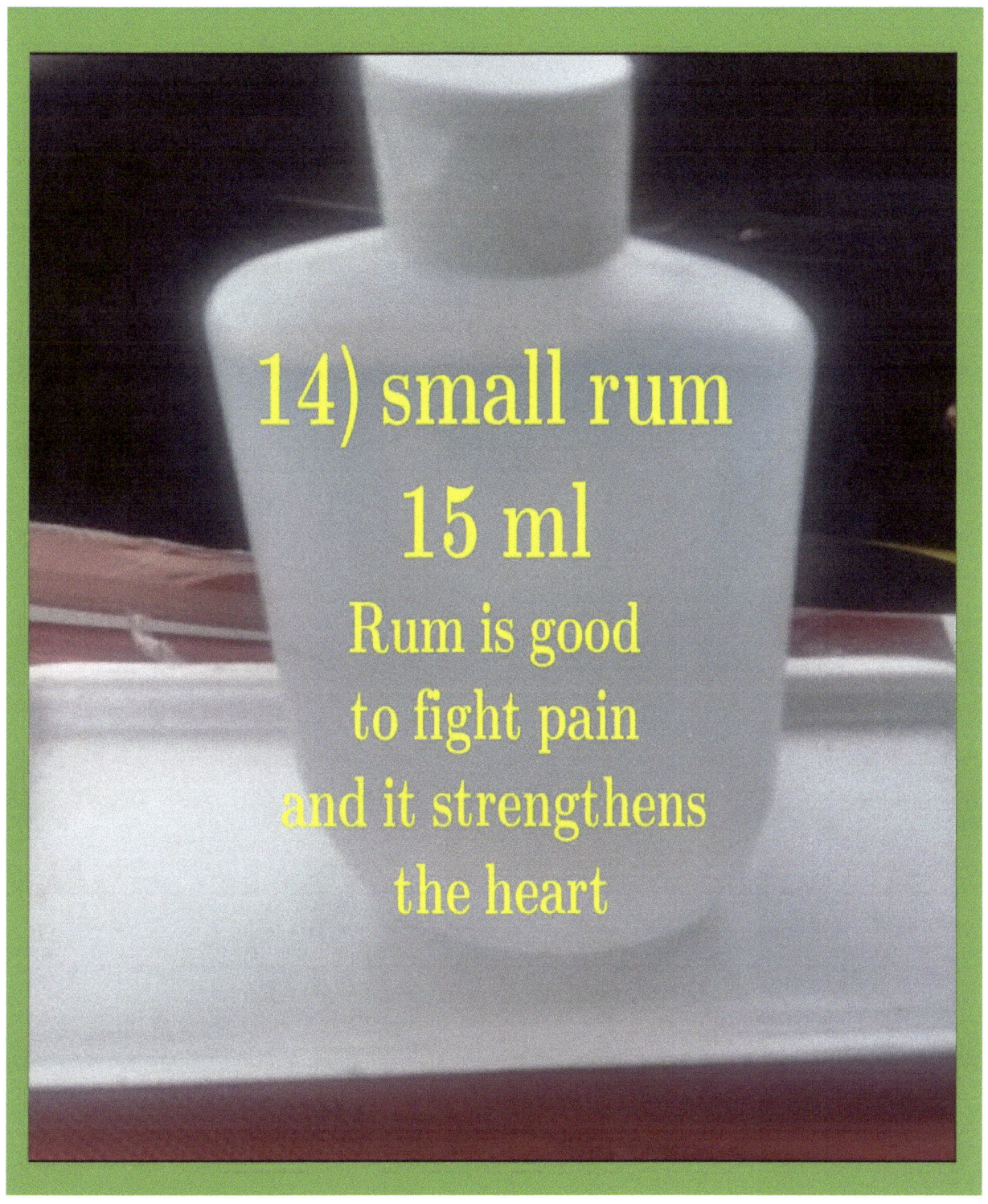
14) small rum 15 ml
Rum is good to fight pain and it strengthens the heart

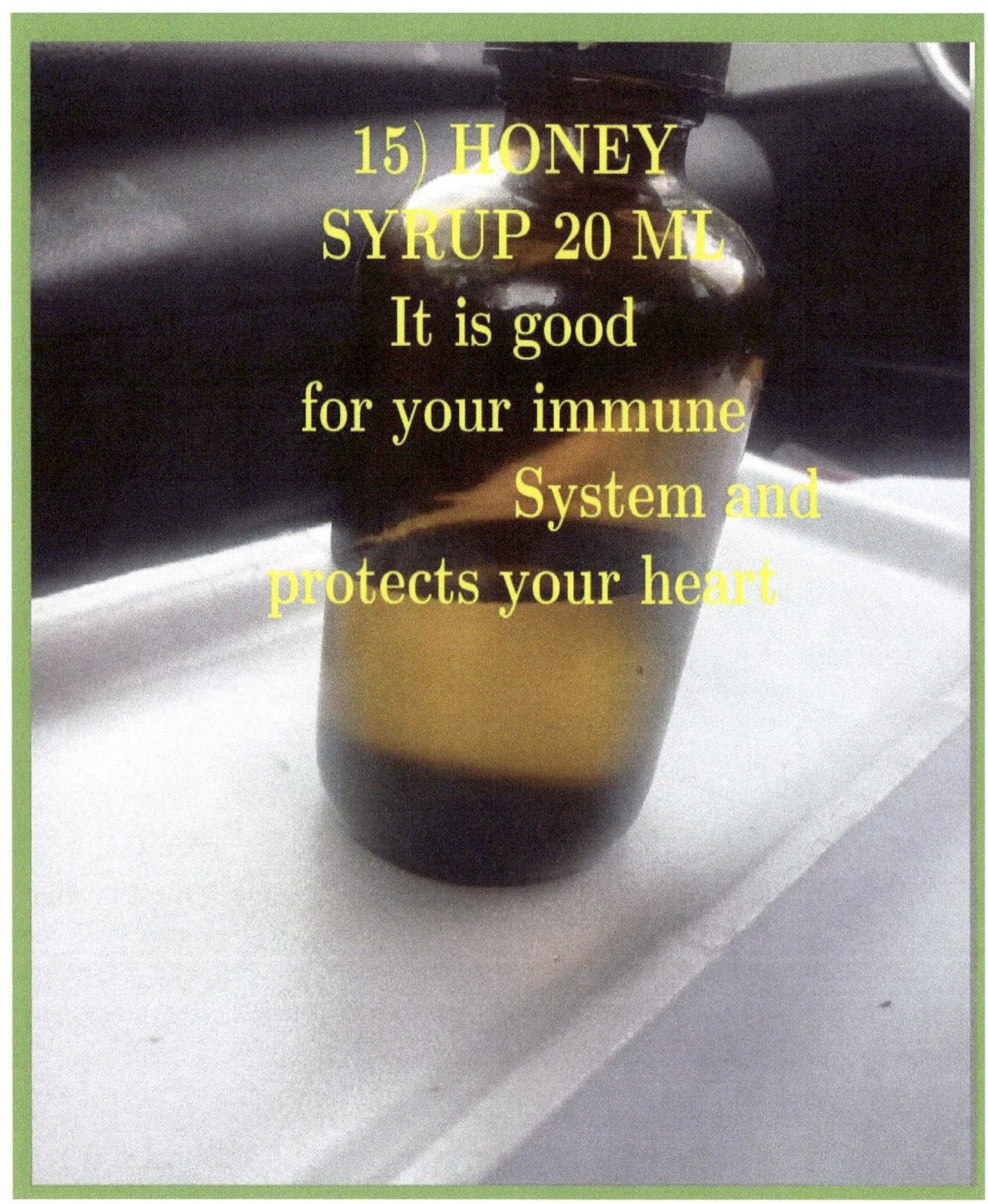

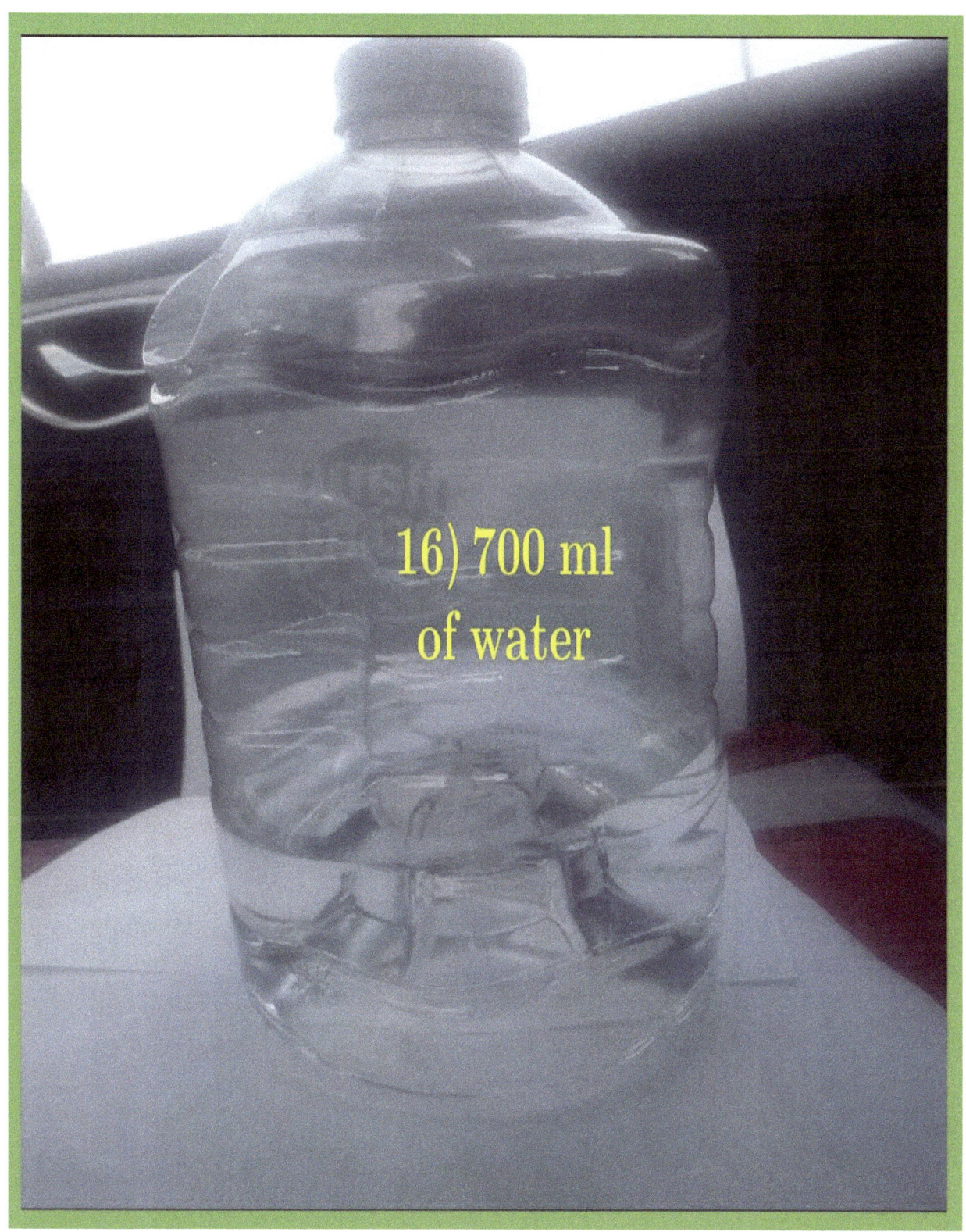

You put them all in a pot. But do not forget you don't have to peel the oranges and lemons; you cut them and add them to boil with all the skin in the syrup. You will cover the pan and let it boil. Let the syrup boil for 15 minutes. After 15 minutes you take down the syrup and pour it into a sieve and put it in a 750 ml bottle and start giving the patient the syrup. The syrup, the bitter water mixed with the tetracycline are the 3 big soldiers that will attack the coronavirus.

7- What foods should patients eat every day? Should the patient drink juice?

Do not forget that corona reaches the entire body of the patient and the patient has no appetite and does not taste food and does not smell, that means you have to encourage him to eat.

In the morning you can give him a nice bowl of soup. Put watercress in it, put bananas and a little meat in it because of the big medicine he is taking. After drinking the soup, give him a small roasted herring and a piece of bread to quench his thirst.

At noon, make a little bean sauce with some vegetables. Do not forget to give the patient a little meat because of the pill to drink.

In the evening you can give him a little broth and meat.

Should the patient drink juice?

No if you give him juice, he will not be interested in drinking the mixed bitter water because he will no longer be thirsty. You may kill the patient without knowing.

Do not forget you need to kill the virus the juice can't do that job, only the mixed bitter water can do that job. After healing, the patient is free to drink whatever he wants.

8- Castor oil: the role of the castor oil. Which side of the patient's body should you pass it to?

Corona often gives the patient a high fever and a runny nose. When this happens, you put the oil through the forehead of the patient and in the middle of the head and you take your finger dipped in the oil and you put your finger inside the patient's nose.

You are doing this in the morning, you are doing it at noon, and you are doing it at night.

9 -Vicks: the role of the Vicks. Which side should you pass it to?

As you use the castor oil, you do the same with the Vicks because it will help patients breathe.

10- Conclusions and recommendations

My God in Jesus never abandons those He loves. He has always the simplest solutions to the most complicated problems. Often the authorities do not want to accept this solution because this solution is too simple. That is why I ask the kings, the presidents, and the great men say the scientists to be friends of Jesus so that their decisions be inspired by God. I know there are some people who would not like a guy like me to come up with coronavirus solutions, but it is God's work. Now coronavirus is a simple fever. You catch coronavirus, you be healed immediately in 3 days. Governments have put restrictions because they did not have solutions for corona but now there are solutions, restrictions must be taken off. Once all restrictions are lifted and everyone knows what to do when they get corona there will be no more coronavirus.

Here are some recommendations:

1) The Author is a Coronavirus survivor; he thinks fit to share his experience to the whole world to stop counting deaths. His book is not a substitute of the governmental recommendations and the medical advice of your doctor

2) for children and for all newly cached adult coronavirus, antibiotics are not necessary. They take only the bitter water mixed and the syrup. The antibiotics in this book are recommended if the patient have an acute fever, the patient can't stand up and the coronavirus reaches a level of serious infection.

3) A caregiver is advised to take the same medication as the patient. A caregiver can take only the bitter water mixed and the sirup syrup.

4) Even if the government does not adopt this book, even if the world health organization does not adopt this document, if you know a person with a dying corona, let him know this book as soon as possible in order to save his life.